TINY RITUALS

108 Poems to Remember Ourselves as Holy, Whole, and Wise

Amber Campion

ISBN: 9798884032835

tender, wild, messy human...*this* is for you.

A NOTE FROM THE AUTHOR

Tiny Rituals didn't start out as a book. It was simply a solution to create a stress-free way for me to get back to something that was once very meaningful to me as a child, *writing poetry.*

It was early 2020 when I found myself longing to write, simply for the sake of writing. Not for a newsletter, or a blog post, or an article, but writing - only for the joy and peace of it.

So I started a no pressure practice of writing 2-3 times a week for 15-30 minutes, and I called these writing blocks, *tiny rituals.*

The only rule for this writing time was -
NO JUDGMENT ALLOWED.

It felt amazing! I didn't edit myself as I was writing, or even when the allotted time was up. The 'great editor' was off duty during these sessions and it felt incredibly freeing.

As time passed, I continued to write, but even the structure of 2-3x's a week faded in and out. I'd hear my inner critic (I call it the *itty bitty shitty committee*) having all sorts of judgments about that, and then I'd have to remind myself that my tiny ritual was not about anything other than joy and peace.

That joy and peace eventually became *a remembering*, which is translated into a journey of 'five books' -

the remembrance of **breaking**, the remembrance of **healing**, the remembrance of **breath**, the remembrance of **presence**, and the remembrance of **self-love**.

These tiny rituals started to feel like a deep spiritual healing. They felt, *I felt* - holy, whole, and wise. In tiny vignettes, there was a story naturally unfolding, the story of me. But more so, a story of the complexity and awe of the human heart. This book holds tiny pieces of not just me, but of all of us.

It was during these tiny rituals that I began to understand, in my bones, that writing (without strict agenda or judgment) is a beautiful and deep embodiment practice. It's not often we humans let ourselves have the luxury of so much space and exploration in our voices, that when we do experience it, it's extraordinarily liberating. My favorite definition for embodiment is *'to be deeply present to direct experience.'* And that is what this practice (these words) offered to me and the place I hope it takes you as well.

Over time I started to notice my poetry could be related to the dharma (purposeful) talks I would give in my yoga classes. I remember the first time I read one of my poems at the end of my class while the students were in Savasana. I felt nervous, but I also felt *wide.*

I started sharing my poems more in class and in other places here and there (women's circles, on social media, in a newsletter). Students would come up to me crying after class, telling me how moved they were by my poem. I started being asked if I could send a copy of this poem or that poem, so they could read them in their yoga classes or women's circles. People would say,

"I need to send this to my mom, or my best friend, or my partner going through a hard time."

And with that, I realized, ironically, this tiny ritual of mine had blossomed into something more than just a remembering *for me*. It had become a remembering for others, as well.

I knew immediately that if I was going to move forward with turning these tiny rituals into a tiny book, I still wanted to stay true to the practice - no pressure, no timelines, no agendas, and certainly no judgment. My only goal was to accumulate 108 pieces of writing for the book, which is a sacred number in yoga (this landed for me as it was many of my yoga students who inspired me to share my poetry more - *thank you!*).

And now, 4-years in the making (not making), **Tiny Rituals** is complete (and never complete). All I really hope for is that you find some semblance of *remembering* as you move through these pages. There is so much joy and peace to be found there.

contents

Table of Contents

CLOSING WORDS...123

BOOK ONE:

The Remembrance of Breaking

and grandma said matter-of-factly,
yet with a kind knowing in her eyes,
'darling, broken crayons can still color.'

majesty in our broken parts

the stars in the sky
look like tiny cracks in the universe,
reminding us
that our majesty can be found
in our broken parts.

the lie we've been told

it's a lie we've been told,
that broken is wrong, unworthy, useless.
that it's better to swallow the illusion of perfection
and believe that wounding is a flaw of the few.
better to hide when you hurt and cover your scars
with armor made of makeup and busy schedules.
it's a lie we've been told, so that we don't *see*
the light seeping through the cracks,
the jagged edges, the shattered spots
that were never meant to break us,
but rather, break us
open

broken, *open*

know this -
life did not simply break you.
it broke you, *open*.
and now the world can not look away
from the luminosity that shines through
the shattered parts.

how many times

how many times have you
discounted your own experience
to preserve someone else's?
how many times have you said,
"it's fine. i'm fine."
when it really wasn't.
when *you* really weren't.

when change asks us to break our *own* heart

in the center of myself
there is a question so painful
that i can not bear to visit it
for more than a few moments at a time,
because i fear *the answer.*

i fear it will turn my world upside down
and burn it to the ground.
i fear it will take all the hope out of me
in one life changing, punch to the gut.
i fear it will remove the earth from under my feet
and fill my eyes with a tsunami so powerful,
it will certainly drown me in a flood of sorrow.

i fear this question so deeply
because it is mine and mine alone
to answer,
which means if it *is* what i fear…

i will be the one who has to break my *own* heart.

on feeling lost

there is a fragile feeling at my very center
- *the core* of who i am.
an uncertainty tugging
like tension in the taut mouth
of someone with debilitating self-doubt.
worries seem to devour me
overwhelm has the power to bury me.
lost, in a way that does not feel free
- a *hungry wolf* sort of lost.
i look forward and all i can see
is an overgrown pathway,
uncleared, rugged.
i *know* i must move forward into this terrain
afraid, my mind becomes evermore foggy.
in a way, i feel *forgotten,*
or like I have forgotten, *myself.*
and in these moments,
life feels like *too much*
yet, at the same time,
not enough.

a letter to loneliness

dear loneliness,
i'm afraid of you.

i fear the solitude will swallow me whole
and the sadness will be a grief i cannot bear to hold;
holding me stuck in the stomach of bottomless emotions

i wonder,
when you look into my eyes,
do you hear the silence in my heart?
do you know what it feels like to be consumed
by the ocean and rocky edges of depression
to feel the hollowness of being isolated,
unseen, an outsider
strapped in by heavy boots sunken into muddy waters
when i'm standing under the night's sky
feeling as though all hope is lost,
i wonder,

who can hear me?

longing

here i am
burning body and tender heart
awaiting the misty light
that seems to always be
just over the horizon of *tomorrow*.
both hopeful and exhausted
trusting and frightened
wavering and resolute
each night i release the weight of another day,
like a heavy backpack dropping off my aching shoulders
and pray to the 'light of tomorrow' that one day
it will be here,
today.

if this falls apart, so will i (the lie my mind tells me)

i look at my calendar, so organized and well planned out
from self care,
to reverse engineered planning sessions,
to time with loved ones.
truly, a hustler's masterpiece!
i scan it over and over again,
with pride and a feeling of authority.
i keep scanning it,
seeing if there are any tiny refinements i can tweak.
more white space, maybe?
are the orange 'exercise' blocks
in balance with the yellow 'self-care' blocks?
hm, creative time for the sake of creative time,
have i scheduled that in?
what color should that be?
and suddenly, deep in my gut, i realize
the illusion of *control* that i've created
in the form of colored coded time blocks.
and now, i feel so clearly
the underlying, quills raised, overwhelm
driving the mirage of finely structured order.
i take a slow breath and at the close of my exhale
i hear the voice in the background of my mind
a sort of consistent and constant anxiety that whispers,
"if this falls apart, so will you."

where and when did this become 'normal'

my mind is achy with pressure
my heart is both heavy and actively pacing
shackled and restless
the lists
the 'to do's'
the balancing act of life
i feel stuck in my head
watching my body on auto-pilot
through two pinholes called eyes
oh! the lies
of chasing success
the cost - endless stress
a daily cup of perfectionism
a weekly dose of procrastination
a silent judgment incessantly lingers in the air
nothing is good enough (including myself)
where and when did this become 'normal'
i want to scream the frustration out of my bones
i want to dance violently
until the anger is weeping from my skin
i want to shake my hands open,
surrendering, once and for all,
my need for safety in the form of control

mis-shaped souls

she believed that her past shaped her.
the pear-shaped weight on her hips
the saddlebags and cellulite on her thighs
the self-given scars on her arms.
she believed that she was broken, at *the core*,
for the longest time
and felt her *mis-shaped soul* would never
find a place in this world.
then, one day she traveled beyond
the borders of familiarity
and met, one by one, other mis-shaped souls
broken at the seams, cracked here and there,
rough around the edges
yet what she noticed was
all the beauty and light
that shined so brightly through those places,
that the world had called broken.

a gratitude letter:
to the 'tough stuff' that made me grow

to death and loss, thank you for reminding me to not
take the love in my heart for any moment or any person,
for granted. thank you for reminding me to hug fiercely
and often, and to look those i care for in the eyes and tell
them what i know they must know, but i must never be
so naive to ever stop saying it - *"i love you."* and to say
it every time, with a tender presence, as if it were going
to be the last time, because you have taught me that one
day - it will be.

to sickness and injury, thank you for reminding me that
my body is a temple and i will be better off to treat this
holy vessel with reverence and deep care. thank you for
showing me that my most valuable commodity is my
health and that every breath i take, *full and alive*, is the
most precious gift i will ever know. thank you to the
bones that carry me, the muscles that move me, and the
skin that holds me. for i now know, that the moment it
can no longer carry me, move me, and hold me - i will
truly appreciate just how *exquisite* this body really was.

to heartbreak and longing, thank you for reminding me
that love is *everything*. it's the dark and the light, the
pain and the pleasure, the beauty and the brutality. thank
you for showing me how extraordinary and grand my
love really is and for breaking my armor open, again and
again, so more and more light could come through.

to confusion and doubt, thank you for not only reminding me, but *insisting*, that i look deeper. thank you for showing me that through the *question*, i'm being invited into a *quest*. And that this awkward journey is not so much about discovering *the one* right answer or path, but rather, it's about being willing to do things differently than i've ever done them before, so i can know my own soul, better than i've ever known it before.

to aging and change, thank you for reminding me of my own humanity. but mostly, thank you for giving me a life *long enough* to bear witness to lines becoming etched on my face and short, white, strangely shaped hairs poking out from the top of my head. thank you for giving me the years to know not just knowledge, but *wisdom* - the kind of knowing that understands it would be wise to not only accept, but *pray* that i get to be around to witness many more lines and gray hairs in this lifetime.

to my darkness and brokenness, thank you for connecting me to the beating heart of this world and to the wholeness that was *always, already* there. thank you for showing me that you were never here to hurt, only to heal.

BOOK TWO:

The Remembrance of Healing

and the *he*artist knew in her bones what you must do
with this gift and said,
'go into the dark and make light.'

it doesn't fit anymore

i was trying to put my armor on today,
but then i realized it doesn't fit anymore.
so i entered the world, *tenderly*
and discovered how truly brave i really am.

an ode to being courageous

i don't want to be fearless
i want to be *courageous*
so i'll be sure to pack
my *heart's wisdom*
for the journey ahead

a burning heart

i know sometimes the fire in your heart
burns almost unbearable.
but you were made *this bright*,
so you could be a lantern
shining *a light*
in the darkness

the knowing in your bones

they'll tell you to leap and the net will appear
but i'll tell you the *truth*, my dear.
there is no net, there never was and never will be.
there is only your faith
your devotion
your willingness to get it wrong.
because deep down you know
in the pulsing of your bones
that you rather spend a lifetime 'getting it wrong'
than live the life that has been laid out before you
meant to dry you out, bones cracked brittle
so you can't hear *deep* anymore.
living life half-mast or living life full-out
they both will have their challenges
so you reach, *even leap* - for grace.
moving towards and facing fear
understanding that there are no promises here,
only a brave journey into the unknown.
and what keeps you going is this knowing
in your bones
that while you may crash and fall
you also suspect
that you may spread your wings
and fly.

advice for when the mind feels full

when the mind is full and the heart feels heavy…
empty out.
s*hake* on the earth
s*plash* upon the water
s*cream* into the wind
br*eathe* fierceness like the fire
when the mind is full and the heart feels heavy…
empty out.

shake it out

you are
undeniable
irresistible
a body full
of starlight and moonbeams
a projection of the highest esteem
so when in doubt
and darling, at times you will
simply, shake it out
shake it out
shake it out
shake out the tears
the fears
the pent-up rage
disengage
from the adversity
of uncertainty
and remember
you are a creation
of improbability
made from a million
impossibilities.

come soothing, not solving

come *soothing,* not solving
because the voice of how things *could be,*
whispers gently.
it does not come to fix and solve, manage and absolve
it simply opens its arms and soothes, *reverently.*
come *soothing,* not solving
because the voice of how things could be, *trusts*
that once you feel safe and seen, loved and serene
you'll know exactly
what to do,
where to go,
and how to say
what you *must.*

meeting my inner grumpy with compassion

when i'm grumpy,
my eyebrows speak,
instead of my mouth -
they draw in and down, furrowing in disapproval.
'in what?, ' you may wonder.
that's the thing -
grumpy never knows what it's upset over
and why it complains
(or at least that's what it mumbles)
it simply builds a wall of angst against the world,
laying down eggshells wherever it goes.
i suspect grumpy needs space
and tender understanding,
but just doesn't have the words for it in the moment.
i'll remember that,
next time grumpy visits.

reflection on healing

there was a time when i focused on my pain, your pain,
all the pain.
sadness filled my belly, swelling it red hot
with desperation.
i *know* pain, but I also know hope -
the light that peeks through the door
after a night of darkness,
that seems to last longer than the last lie i told myself,
before i was brave enough to seek the truth.
hope - it's under the door again, teaching me to wonder.
there are three humming birds that once visited me -
i was told to listen, *closer.*
and i could hear it - *laugher* - in the tree's
a freedom waiting for me.
now i have something that keeps me safe
even when the darkness finds me in a corner
of my own making.
i have a knowing, a sensing, a feeling
i have been broken - *open.*
there is trust in my blood, like a flowing river
and *i see now,* what my hands are making
and my breath is holding
between the balance of
reaching out
and resting in
my own humanity

healing on the horizon

there is *healing on the horizon*
it is felt in the deep sighs
and witnessed in the tender tears
welling in the collectives eyes
a freedom is calling from within
the spaciousness of possibility
a levity lifting us into action
because hope is not wishing
but rather, *it is walking*
in the direction of a vision
whole bodied and made of a *holy* kind of grief
we march forth
pulling heavy lumber to the edge of the sea
building boats, fires, and futures
for a dream
for a chance
for change

a call to heal

you are a holy temple.
do what you must
to keep your higher Self sovereign
and remember
healing is a rebellious and sacred act
of *embodied* leadership
not just meant for business suits and boardrooms
but a kind of leadership
that speaks through all you do and all you be

heal your body
so you can lead with grace

heal your mind
so you can lead with truth

heal your heart
so you can lead with love

naming it is *everything*

today i named it.

i named the thing that had me wanting
to run away and hide.
pretending i don't care - *wishing*, from a distance,
that i didn't.
that thing that had been holding my sunken, tender heart
in its unrelenting hands.
leaving me exhausted by the notion of *'still'* being *here,*
feeling little, alone, confused, let down.

today i named it.

i called it out from the wild, roaming narratives
that haunt my mind.
i said it so simple and so clear, it landed
like a polaroid - slowly, but surely, coming into focus.
a moment of still silence crept in
and the truth poured *up* my throat
and slid down my tongue like a waterfall.

nothing else was said for many moments
as layers of armor fell from my skin.
then softly, yet like sipping in air for the first time,
in a long time -
these four words freed themselves from my mouth like a
breath of fresh air… *"i finally named it."*

like all wild things

there is something so tenderly wild
about *letting go -*
like watching a tumble weed blow, *you know?*
it was once *attached* from where it came
i wonder if it struggled, held on,
fought to keep things the same.
regardless, like all wild things
it wanders now,
boundless and free.

i remember i'm holy, whole, and wise

i *remember* i'm holy, whole, and wise
when i give myself the dignity
of being in my body,
fully and truly,
even when it's hard.
when i let the softness
and the roughness meet
with reverence *and remember*
this body of mine is not a temptress,
but a *temple.*
when i surrender the moments in life,
even if just for a moment,
that want me to believe it's not safe to be *here.*
and i can again whole-heartedly
remember who i am.
it is here, *embodied*
deeply present to both the beauty and brutality
of my humanness,
that i can look myself in the mirror
and say with certainty,
'yes, you, i can go to bed with you every night.'

part 1: what i will remember, for when i need it most

embodiment is staying present
to the beauty and brutality
of what is/our humanness.
embodiment is unguarded.

tender human,
i see you
and what it takes
to come back to this place,
again and again.

disembodiment is running from,
suppressing, diffcring, ignoring, judging
what is/our humanness.
disembodiment is armored.

tender human,
i see you
and what it takes
to notice you are here,
again and again.

neither place is 'good or bad'…*just human.*

part 2: what i will remember, for when i need it most

i lay here,
armored, *yet again*
i have raveled myself
into a million tight knots
made of should's and judgements,
jealousies and self-doubt.
but this time i let myself breathe.
this time i *remember*
that where i have found myself
is not 'good or bad'
it's just *human.*
and *this,*
makes all the difference.

letting go and being seen

you do not need to prove your worthiness,
displayed like trophies across a dusty shelf
to get approval.
you do not need to push forward,
like a soldier on the battlefield,
to be enough.
you do not need to prostrate yourself
before the feet of humans,
to belong.
you only need to let your long held armor
fall from your tender heart,
and let the light of your humanity
be seen.

observing

observing - that has been home for me lately.
sitting back, more than pushing forward.
less on the calendar, more time in bed.
the stillness has me feeling, *more.*
bearing witness to an old familiar 'hum'
in the background of my mind.
an overwhelming feeling like 'falling behind'
or getting 'lost in the light of others.'
it's intoxicating and scratches at me to dress
in an armor made of metal clad 'shoulds'
and rawhide leather 'worry.'
i feel it rise in my throat,
like being choked by hands from within.
and yet, i'm able to take a breath.
i'm able to relax my shoulders.
i'm able to listen to the clamor of my own making
without breaking into a sweat,
and riding off into the wind
with only the indirect marching orders
from an inner phantom.
instead, i watch this all unfolding in me,
like watching a movie from the *inside*, out.
captivated, emotional, yet this time…

i know i'm entirely safe and holding the remote.

guilt-free self-care

self-care today was allowing myself
to stay in bed until 8am.
it wasn't so much the sleeping in
that felt so nourishing and needed,
but more so, that I did it,
 guilt-free.

note to self:
spend more time savoring life - *guilt-free*

**a word about self-doubt
(from someone who knows it well)**

and your doubt can become
like a dimmer switch in your heart
lowering the light of possibility
if you let yourself forget,
that doubt,
is just *one* voice.

self-doubt meets self-trust

self-doubt, i'm onto you…
you fool me into thinking
that you're simply a little 'worry' visiting.
your entrance begins smooth and unassuming
as if the distress is no more than a temporary aid
to keep me on my toes -
but you're more than that.
you visit not only when i question choices,
but when i question my *worth*
you love to show up when i feel
hallowed, tired, discouraged
you relish in my disbelief and the secret panic inside
only intensifies your presence.
before i know it, i am captivated by you
imprisoned in my own head,
quivering in endless stories of 'not enough.'
i see now, that this is where you'd like me to live forever
another prized soul for your taking.
but i will not be fooled so easily
for my dreams are born of tougher things
and i have taken on an ally that you can not defeat -
self-trust

learning to trust yourself

those moments when you doubt yourself
you doubt your worth
you doubt you'll find your way back, *or at all*
those moments feel like eternity, wrapped in eternity
like a delicate, yet reckless
tangled gold chain necklace
you wonder, *"can this ever be undone?"*
then patience whispers…
"slowly, slowly, darling. walk, don't run."
and i suspect
this is how all knotted up things
eventually become free.

shedding skin

a gentle, caring reminder…

not all change needs to be a walk through the fire;
a battle in the field of existence.
you need not burn yourself to the ground,
every time you shed a skin.

can you release in a way that is nurturing
and holds you softly,
so you can experience,
not just the fear, loss, and grief,
but the *beauty* of change.

can you let yourself move on and forward
with dignity and self-respect?

sacred change

the tenderness of growth
requires us to hold (ourselves and others) with care.
this is how breakdowns can not help but to blossom -
into breakthroughs

strength in your softness

there is so much strength
in your softness

yet, the world will teach you
vulnerability is weakness
that you must toughen up
create a shell around you -
this way you'll be protected…
from life

yet, we forget
that softness,
like water gliding through rock beds
has the power to shape shift
even the toughest surfaces,
breaking down stone and creating worlds,
patiently

the armor, your heart, and you

and the armor that shouted, *"i'm not vulnerable!"*
was slowly removed.
and it was stunningly beautiful to witness.
my heart whispered,
'thank you for allowing me to see you.'
and the one beneath the armor unexpectedly replied,
"no one ever sees me. thank YOU."

listening to the body

i've got tired bones
a feeling of heavy
water weighted blankets
wrapped around me
from head to toe

you know that kind of tiredness?
the kind that penetrates you right down
to your weary bones.

it's a message, you know.
because when the bones start speakin'
the soul is singin'...*the blues.*

so i took a nap today.
woke up and wrote this…

'i'm listening now, dear body. i'm listening.'

between the shadow & the light

work hard. play hard.
design every moment to be impeccable.
this exhausting mentality, conditioned impracticality
is revered and placed upon a golden pedestal.
the addiction to more, the longing for less.
we battle the polarity between the 'no' and the 'yes.'
again and again, we go until we can't
then we rest, bone-weary
arms thrown up in a tear-drenched chant.
surrendered.
only now do we listen for that familiar call home
a perfect flow, like honeycomb
weaving in resonate tone.
so radiant. so peaceful.
so we promise ourself this time will be different
this time i won't jump into the raging current
or lose myself, atrophied and wind burnt.
this time…
i'll slow tango with 'no,' gently caress the 'yes.'
i'll make it my devoted quest
to meet the moment,
and *lean*
into the spaces that rest…
between.

the awakening

a door opens.
i step through
and for the first time,
i truly *see*.

i see all the fears
all the stories
all the doubt
that kept me from stepping through
a thousand times before.

i see it all, and yet, it feels so distant.
like i've gone on a long, *long* journey
to take *a single* step forward.

and while this step may seem insignificant
on the outside,
i know the inward mountains i've climbed
and the falls i've risked,
all so i could step through
and see this familiar place,
as if for the first time.

the sacred why

and we hold on
for all the light
we can not *yet* see

BOOK THREE:

The Remembrance of Breath

and the wind whispered,
'who do you breathe the deepest with? go there.'

breathe with your whole body

you are a river of infinite channels
a holy earth vessel of loamy soil
and waves of time travel
an exquisite *masterpiece* - a *piece* of the *master*
made of bits and pieces of stardust
from ancient supernovas
y*ou* are an intimate part of the *whole* universe
undeniably *someone*, because you are the *sum of one*
a portal of cosmic connection
a doorway to possibility
a rare chance in time and space
from the tips of your toes
to the top of your head
from the inside, *out*
and the outside, *in*
y*ou are life force energy*
galaxies of prana exist within you
tingling, rippling, waving, spiraling through you
reminding you that you are inherently
holy, whole, and wise.
so the next time you take a breath
breathe with your *whole body*
and feel your ancestors,
the moonbeams and solar flares,
lighting you up and whispering to you,
"you were always enough."

the way to inspiration

words have history,
explore them
and you'll discover
ancient *rememberings* and remedies.
for instance
the word *inspiration*
comes from the latin root,
inspiratus or *inspirare*
it essentially means,
'breathe life into' or *'to infuse with (life).'*
this tells us
that for as long as time
has been recorded,
the way to inspiration
has always been
to breathe.

lay it down and breathe

if it feels heavy - *lay it down*
your worries, your worst-case scenarios,
your addictions to drama, to pain, to overwhelm
lay. it. down.
let yourself free from the mind traps
that use your imagination to spark a flame called 'fear'
locking into your gut like a gnarly rotted root.
conjure another possibility
dare to ignite a flame called 'love'
dancing you open along the waters of wonder
tickling your curiosity into care; you're free to go there.
the ticket is that... *you must breathe*
and if the temptations of worry
are a force bigger than your devotion to live in love
i encourage you to *pray, shake, chant*
your way to liberation
because if you have truly come to a crossroad
called 'no choice'
then worry will not help.
and if there is a chance of other paths
then still, worry will not aid you
so give yourself reprieve.
lay down the brutal burdens of your imagination
lay down the weight of a story you can not bear
lay down the heavy lifting of illusion
and breathe sister. breathe, brother.
breathe.

notice what you notice, feel what you feel

simply *arriving*
is the hardest part -
not just to the yoga mat
or in the body,
but *within.*
withstanding the parts of us
that feel hooked on distraction
keeping us arms distance
from presence and peace of mind.
so we land in the moment
by committing to the only thing we can -
the breath
and the devotion to, again and again,
notice what we are noticing
and feel what we are feeling
is no small practice,
in a world that would prefer us distracted
but rather,
an act of *holy* rebellion

winds of change

when the winds of change are felt upon your skin
it may feel like pieces of your life are being removed.
in those moments, the wind is *reminding you*
that strength can be found in the things we can't see,
yet certainly can *feel.*
it's reminding you to breathe.

you are like the wind

as i stood on a mountain
that took half a lifetime to climb
and as the wind blew across my face
and through my hair
i closed my eyes and opened my heart
i took a slow breath, and i heard it!
the wind singing…

*'wild thing - you are like me, you have always been free -
infinite, ever-changing, and utterly incapable of being
caged.'*

a reminder from the breath

breathe into the *deep end* of your life
away from the shallow false safety of illusions.
your breath is a reminder of the *fullness* of who you are -
with every inhale and every exhale,
the life force of ancestors tingles upon your sacred skin.
wholeness can be restored here
and *a remembering*
that you are nothing short of *holy*.

—*lovingly, the breath*

wonder of the breath

who would've thought
that whole galaxies of energy
could be felt.
that portals of potential
could be met.
that the expanse of eros
could be channeled.
that pain and peace
could become one.
that doubt
could alchemize into wonder
and fear
could fade into love.
all within -
the breath.

for questions we can not answer

*how do we hold ourselves up
when the weight feels larger than us?*

*how do we seek the light
when we stand in the shadow?*

*how do we connect with resiliency
when we're in the center of the wreckage?*

first, we stop asking *how.*

'how' will hold us hostage in a suffering
made of impossible questions to answer.
it will bury us in endless loops
of worry, doubt, indecision, and mistrust.

rather, inquire into *'why,' 'what,'* or, at times, *'when'*
then, the answer will emerge from your heart,
rather than your head.

**'why' do you hold yourself up
when the weight feels larger than you?**

breathe and feel the answer in your body.
feel the pulsing of your purpose
in the center of your being

**'what' brings in the light
when you stand in the shadow?**

breathe and feel the answer in your body.
feel the pulsing of your practice
in the center of your being

'when' *do you connect with resiliency?*
here, the second part *is* your answer...

'when you're in the center of the wreckage'

you are living poetry

you are more than your memories
you are living, *breathing* poetry
a true telling of humanity
so, with every breath of life you breathe,
remember, you are symbolically writing poetry.
now, with that being clear,
please do so,
with the deepest reverence
and care.

a prayer for surrender (ishvara pranidhana)

no matter the outcome of this journey…
help me to see my life through eyes of love
guide me to trust my path and what i'm here to do
support me to take the *next* right step, without hesitation
remind me to slow down
and see how far i've already come
and most importantly, grant me the gift of forgiveness,
so that i may be free when i breathe my last breath

Om shanti, shanti, shanti
Om peace, peace, peace

BOOK FOUR:

The Remembrance of Presence

'how does one slow down time?' asked the busy adult.
and the precocious child answered, *'savor more.'*

what presence taught me

when things are easy, *soften.*
when things are hard, *soften more.*

presence is medicine

this right *here*
right *now* moment
is *your life*.
it's your dreams, your future memories,
your contribution in time.
it's the direction, the path, the perspective
you're laying down as a guide.
and while there will be things you can not define
you do get to choose if those tracks
will be narrow or wide.
so till the soil of this moment, and the next
with *curiosity*, rather than assumptions
patience, rather than frustration
deep care, rather than avoidance
love, rather than fear
and *presence* will become medicine of the highest order
a balm soothing your wounds
and wooing your heart warrior
a sanctuary with no borders
this right *here*
right *now* moment
is *your life*.

the most powerful thing you have

tune into the most powerful thing you have -
the power of *your attention* in the present moment.
truth lives here,
and the more *here* you are,
the more expanded your life becomes.

the messenger of presence

there's a hummingbird that lives in my heart
hum, humming to the beat of my feet,
creating a determined path
reminding me, to enjoy it *all*,
as too quickly, time will pass.
it sips nectar from the bitter sweetness of my existence
reminding me, *to savor,* to integrate,
and to honor the reminiscence.
and in the midst of all my human
brewing, doing, and accruing,
it never ceases to buzz in patterns
boundless, wild, and free
reminding me, what *my soul* came here to be.

taking counsel in your unbound heart

there is a place
in the center of your *unbound* heart
that is still, vulnerable, and flawless.
it pays *true attention* to your life
noticing compassionately
habit energies and narratives
that spin in your mind like an old record
catching the fine groove of a scratch
over and over and over, again.
dare to give your heart's wisdom
a seat at the table
taking counsel from the untethered
field of deeper knowing.
it is *here*
you will find the kind of strength
that is soft and open
inviting you to truly know,
your *Self*

savoring the right now moments

savoring the *right now* moments
is the most courageous practice,
the most glorious prayer.
to stay present within both the beauty
and brutality of impermanence
is an awakening into a surrender of the *deepest depths*.
to know, *in your bones*, that this life will pass us all by
is opening to an unshakable aliveness in the face
of eternal rest.
to see the world today,
as if you will not be dancing in it tomorrow
allows for the senses to come alive - *tender. raw. radiant.*
all the things of this world come into view,
yet *slowly, slowly, slowly*
and with an unutterable peace and presence
holding you in this moments season
like water seeping from the cracks
of a once armored life,
the neurosis fade
and all that is left is reverence and love,
without any apparent reason.
yet you *now* know - it's all there ever was.
everything else was an illusion.

mindfulness broken down (in a minute)

9:09am:
time - it races by
well, that's what they say, *anyway.*

yet i have another story to tell
it's a slow motion kind of potion
that slithers from the center of your core
and can make your spirit soar.
to enter, take a deliberate breath
okay, maybe a few more - *slowly, slowly* now
begin to feel your truth, *within.*

sensation rises
maybe an ache or a chill on your skin
you look down and see your hands, *really* see them
the lines, the life, the resemblance to your kin

then you notice laughter from across the room
'*she's so present,*'
(hmm, where did that thought come from?)
*y*ou're not sure, but it seems to pull you closer to a kind
of truth, *within.*

you never noticed before how tender his smile was
he's shy, yet fierce. you can see him *clearly* now.
'*remember this,*'
(hmm, where did that thought come from?)
again, you're not quite sure, but it seems to pull you
closer to a kind
of truth, *within.*

a sip of water - you can taste the nourishment
upon your lips.
'thank-you, thank-you, thank-you'
(hmm, where did that thought come from?)
you're beginning to get it, this connection to a kind
of truth, *within*
that seems to slow life down enough to actually,
witness it.

9:10am:
time - it races by
well, that's what they say, *anyway.*

an invitation to un-complicate things

the ego (aka 'the great editor')
makes everything so messy
telling us to go this way and that way
do this, do that, do more, do better!
mindfulness is the practice of *un-complicating things.*
it invites us into the present moment,
without the 'great editor'
judging and nit picking our every move.

gratitude

there is a place we can all go
to refill what has been depleted -
the birds, the sun
the changing colors of a new season
the softness of a flowing creek
the smell of rain, the sound of thunder
the joy heard between the branches of a tree
the moonlight flirting with each flickering star
look, and you'll agree, it's so clear to see
the endless dew-drops of awe and wonder
teaching us that a grateful heart is not a privilege.
but rather, *a practice*, of noticing all the beauty
that exists right *here.*

all that matters

today, as i woke up,
a *pure* stillness captured me.
time stood still as i noticed
shadows from the branches outside,
dancing on my wall.
in that moment,
it was so clear to me
that the simplicity
of this moment,
was all that mattered.

what we do

again, and again, and again
the heart will be broken wide open
and the soul will feel it's losing its voice.
in those moments, *surrender to stillness.*
in that space, your heart and soul can mend
and rise from the ashes
again, and again, and again.

an impenetrable softness

there's an *impenetrable* softness
that exists within
a space that knows how to gently hold
the weight of things therein
as tender as the rising and falling of a baby's breath
or holding another's hand, towards the walk to death
oh yes! there is a place *within*
a space that knows how to gently hold
the weight of things that cut-in
and like the push and pull of a slow tango
you slowly learn how to dance with both the light
and *the shadow*

there is a space inside

there is a space inside
go there.
dare to slowly peel back the layers -
the doubt
the agitation
the anger
the grief
move beyond the shallow end of your life
into the deep, deep end
to begin again,
here.
where mystery and freedom
await you.

song of the body

listen closer and you'll hear it
a whisper at first,
like wind gently blowing through leaves
or a soft kiss at the nape of your neck.
you must slow down to align with it's rhythm
you must be *present* to witness it's majesty
you must be home, *in your bones*, to know it's wisdom.
the *song* of the body moves through your spine
like the breath through a woodwind instrument
as clear as crystalline
rocking back and forth in harmony with humanity
fingers like keyboards reaching for resonance
the ribcage resounding in melodic notes
the heartbeat thumping with the sweetness
of the crescendo and decrescendo
of your breath.
at times, the cadence is spirited and bold
then some measures, sorrowful and heavy
a few notes dance with the whimsical
and gracefully glide you through a tempo of tranquility
the music enraptures and captures
what words can not -
a poetic understanding
that a world is expressed through and within
the *holy, whole,* and *wise* song of the body

welcome yourself home

in this modern day we live in the routine,
rather than *the ritual*
we value ourselves, like commodities
giving over our hours, our days, our *life*
to a list, to a plan, to a dream - that was never ours
we have forgotten *the sacred,* the ceremony
the tender intentional personal clearing
an opening to *the holy*
the divine light that cracks us open to our 'wild and free'
a welcoming of nature into our bodies
a moment for the mind to reflect
a space for the heart to envision
a gathering of tribe in community,
in unity
the ritual has been lost, to a routine
but it doesn't have to be so
welcome it back
dare to slow down your pace
letting your life catch up to you
and in the ritual, awaken life into the places
that have become like a dull sigh
inviting *your song* back into your bones
and *your truth* back into your heart
and *your tenderness* back into your eyes
and *your strength* back into your soul
welcome it back…
so you can welcome *yourself* home.

the dash

between the date of your birth
and the date of your death,
lies a dash.
that *dash* (-)
insignificant as it may seem
between such momentous dates
as life and death,
is actually of the utmost importance
when you consider its breadth.
that 'simple dash' between birth and death
represents, *your life.*
so the question stands,
what will you do with
your dash?

advice from death

before it's too late -
can we be brave enough
to slow down, pick our heads up
and truly see the beauty in a world
that will not always be ours.

-death (offering purpose)

on stretching ourselves

capacity is the conversation we have
with ourselves and with others,
about what the truth of our 'stretch' looks like
at any given moment.
this is not a set and done kind of conversation,
but rather an on-going inquiry.
stretching, whether literally or figuratively,
requires our *presence*,
not our 'shoulds.'

trade it in for your true self

with every passing year,
you'll come to know that *time*
is your most precious resource,
so sooner than later,
trade in being your *'best'* self
for being your *'true'* self.

BOOK FIVE:

The Remembrance of Self-Love

*'how can i liberate myself
from this relentless self-doubt,'*
pleaded humanity.

And their wise, higher self proclaimed,
*'to trust your tender, knowing he(art) -
keep it wide and wild,
soft and surrendered.
and also,
don't forget your self-loving fucking boundaries.'*

initiation of the small spark

i have given up bigger, better, faster
for shedding, softer, truer.
now i know how to be a light
that doesn't burn me to the ground.

a short essay on self-love and success

it's not bubble baths or big bank accounts -
though both those things are delightful.
it's not affirmations or accolades -
though both those things are helpful.
it's not fancy chocolate
or the number of 'followers' we have -
though both those things can temporarily
fuel the illusion.

self-love and **success** are two words that get thrown
around like dice at a casino. and just like the glowing
lights that draw us into the gamble, we bet our most
precious resource on the game, *our life*.

with such high stakes, i encourage all of us to take a
deeper look into what self-love and success might really
look like *for you*. from what I can tell, they both entail
leaning in enough towards our deepest *soul-level*
longings, that we actually *mess up* along the way. it
seems, despite what we've been told, *perfection* has
nothing to do with our worthiness of love or success.

here's what i've come to know about self-love and
success...

self-love is daring to fail because you love your dreams
so much, *it's worth it.*
success is picking yourself back up, again and again,
stronger each time, wiser, more humble…and *more
human.*

self-love is recognizing that your dreams are worthy of
being so, so much so, that they *must* live, no matter the
outcome.
success is taking the paintbrush into your hand and
beginning before you even know what your first stroke
will be (and *trusting* that the first stroke is not a
reflection of how the last one will turn out).

self-love is recognizing the power in rest and doing what
it takes to get sufficient sleep.
success is doing that - *guilt-free.*

self-love is boundaried, yet curious.
success is following those curiosities.

self-love is being an unrelenting seeker of your *own*
truth.
success is getting that we don't *find* our path, we *create*
it.

self-love is living in ways that others may not
understand.
success is forgiving yourself for that.

self-love is getting intimate with the depths of your fear, the limiting stories you're attached to, and befriending the parts of yourself that you're afraid for others to see.

success is being vulnerable, not having all the answers, and admitting when you're wrong - yet still believing in yourself, through and through.

self-love is suspending self-judgment long enough that another voice can enter - the voice of your *true* Self. **success** is liberating yourself from conventional expectations, and following your unconventional 'crazy' heart…because even though you aren't certain, you suspect that life truly comes alive along the edges of your crazy heart.

begin here

and my heart whispered, *"begin here..."*

where stillness holds you in the sweet nectar of *now*
and the tender truth of your *deep heart* can be heard.
dare to feel your way into those unexplored places
calling you forth -
feel the textures of its walls, the patterns and curves
notice the colors, both faded and vibrant
let the *unfamiliar* slowly become a warm embrace
and trust this stranger, called the unknown,
will soon be anything but.

it starts with you

imagine if all people
welcomed you
as you are.
imagine if it started
with you.

- self-love

with love, *boundaries*

support, *yes.*
hold space, *certainly.*
and also remember…
when others repeatedly ask you to carry their weight
when they bring only their wounds to a relationship
you can't expect it to thrive.

- lovingly, your boundaries

no such place as 'perfect'

i wish someone would have told me a long time ago
that there's no such place as 'perfect.'
that i can't work, charm, exercise, or meditate my way
out of *being human.*
so moving forward, i vow to do this for you,
whomever is willing to listen
to let you know in poetry, in song, in story -
the *truth* about life.
and i say this with the most tender love,
in hopes it will soothe the sting
but you must know this, darling
there will be pain.
you can do 'allthethings' to try and erase it away
but the reality is, you live in the space between
tension and tone, dissonance and resonance
this is our human agreement. our school and our church.
our poems, songs, and stories
come from this space between
keeping us tethered to you, to me, to humanity.
so dear one, i'm here to tell you
there is *no* such place as 'perfect,'
yet, when you really get this in your bones
you'll find you've arrived
at another place,
one that *does* exist -
called, *peace of mind.*

an act of holy rebellion

in a world that tells you that your worth
is in choosing to chase bigger, faster, more -
it is surely an act of holy rebellion to decide
you've always been enough,
then slowly drive off in your used suburu,
with your priceless joy and peace of mind.

grace

grace.
my body moves
in search of it.
not the longing kind of search
but a willing and curious kind.
by now i have learned
that only in the surrender
and honoring of my pace
can i witness the marvel and majesty of grace.
it begins at the foot step of listening…*closer*
a dancing with the pulsing divinity within
a noticing of the echo - the small, *still* voice
the celestial soul song of a greater knowing
full, *yet spacious* is how it feels
an opening of the heart
upon a soft, yet strong and centered self.
the moment is a precious and holy remembering
in quiet awe, tears well up and stream down my face
as peace washes over me in the simmering of poetry in
grace.

divine feminine

perfection, *meh.*
i would rather this…

a body made of mossy earth
so you can lean against it
when you need to *feel softer*

a heart made of salt water
so you can float in it
when you need to *feel lighter*

a mind made of celestial light
so you can soar in it
when you need to *remember your boundlessness*

- the divine feminine

do you know

do you know that you are *holy, whole, and wise*
from the tips of your toes to the top of your head.

did you know that your bones know how to listen
for answers that your mind can not translate;
and that your hips can simultaneously hold and release
lifetimes of timelines both brutal and beautiful.

are you aware that your hands can bear a thousand
broken hearts simply because of the *one* beating behind
your chest; and that your eyes can see another's soul
when you're brave enough to take off *your own* mask.

as you journey deeper and deeper into yourself,
you will discover that you are not alone,
and never have been.

your inner world is a reflection of *all* of humanity. your
fears and doubts are not so different from others; just as
your hopes and dreams also move across an invisible
thread that reaches a part of everyone, connecting you to
all that is, in the most delicious way - *intrinsically,
deeply, honestly.*

getting to know intimacy

i am intimacy.
i listen to the heart and retrain the brain to see, *truth.*
i am slow and deep, inclusive and real.
i am raw.
i feel like beauty and brutality
i have no discrimination between the two.
life, is what i offer.
i am ritual and ceremony, discomfort and dis-ease.
i am home.
i live in the glint of your eye
and the pulse of your blood.
i have no agenda
other than to expose to you
the fullness, the richness
of *truly* living.
i'm available - the moment the mask is removed.
i stir up fear, but i am not fear itself.
i will wrangle up insecurities
but i am not your self-doubt or loathing.
i am your truth, beneath your humanness
and *the answer*
to your soul's deepest and most vulnerable questions.

catch up to you

dear dreamer,
let me tell you what loving a dream really is.
it's slowing down enough
to let that *wild, tender, beautiful* dream -
catch up to you.

sankalpa

meeting life with intention
is a practice - *a ritual*.
not a plan or a routine.
this can be hard for those of us
who've been conditioned to believe
it's only safe to live within the confines of control
{a tender knowing nod to family drama and trauma}
intention is where we stop reacting to our conditioning
and *start responding*
to our truth

the sacred pause

the sacred pause is an act of self-love.
the body is a river of wisdom - *are you listening to it?*
space. time. reflection -
the world will have you think this is a luxury.
it is not.
it's a necessity.
inward is not a direction, it's *a dimension* -
with breadth and depth.
a place of reverence and re-wilding.
it holds the key to all your questions.
as it's a return, *to love.*
and a *remembering -*
that we are holy, whole, and wise.

embodiment of your own divinity

dear sisters and brothers, queen and kings, gods and
goddesses…

do you know it yet?

your *own* beauty.
your *own* grace.
your *own* dignity.

have you yet *seen yourself,*
through the eyes of the divine?
have you dared to release your armor
and bare yourself naked?
have you been brought to your knees in radiant tears,
by the power of your *own* self-love?

the one true face of myself

over my lifetime,
i have known many faces of myself,
identities that have both held me and held me down.
but i have only known *one* face
that truly reflects the Self - *love*.

the one true face of myself

trust your he(art)

no matter how many times it has been broken (open)
no matter the personal hurts, wounds, lies
you've lived with
no matter the stories, the circumstances,
the justifications
trust your wild, precious, tender he(art)
trust what it wants to create
whether that be
a painting, a poem, a business, a baby, a home
it's *all* a work of art
if it comes from the depths
of your honest, holy heart

on embodiment

open me up
like a rising from my core, through my heart,
up into my throat
not a volcano bubbling up, threatening to erupt.
but rather, like the wings of a bird
fluttering, adapting, daring to take off,
into the wonder of full flight.
my throat speaks to me in sensations that flutter
like wings of a bird
a sort of elder living on the ridges of my soft palate.
when this wise mother comes to me with bird energy
i know she senses my tenderness.
she comes to cleanse my fear of being heard.
not being heard in the straightforward kind of way
but the kind of being heard
that strips you down naked,
un-armors you,
and frees you like a wild bird.

understanding is love's other name

an elder said, *'understanding is love's other name.'*
and i understand this best, when i am *in* my bones
that this body - made of stardust and lovemaking -
knows how to listen, *softly.*
so, i open my heart and let life's tenderness ease its way
into my pores
pouring from a thousand petals,
containing a thousand tears
into the depth of my vessel
so i can truly *understand.*
and like a river flowing
i am set free
by *love.*

poem inspired by a thich nhat hanh quote
"understanding is love's other name."

once and for all (women)

move in a way that lets your body sing it's song
let her roar if she must roar
weep if she must weep
laugh in hysteria, if she must.
let her be as sensual as silk
and as rough as the thorns of rambling roses
let the curves of her thighs
and the rolls of her belly
shake in ecstatic surrender
to the vast harmonies that reside within her flesh.
the stories she can not yet tell
the history she can not yet reconcile
the rising up and the falling down
let her move in a way
that *this* song, once and *for all*,
can beat through and out
can burn from her heart
and drench the pores
so freedom can be felt
once and *for all*
and a song that only your body can sing
can be sung
even if only…*once*
and *for all (women)*.

reflections on taking up space

i take up space
and am told
that's too big
too much
too bold.
so, little by little
i reach
for a possibility
a semblance of credibility
in a patriarchy of fragility
reaching out
tuning in
reaching out
tuning in
reaching out
tuning in
playing these two polarities like a symphony
an orchestration of divine inner harmony
a vulnerable *'yes, and'*
a valiant display
of one who
little by little
reached for something new
and stopped asking for permission
to take up space

rise anyway

in one's lifetime,
so precious and tender,
there will be endless stories of landslides
and sinking ships that will break our hearts.
again and again, our insides will shatter
into tiny fractures and fragments
of sharp, distorted edges.
these become our walls, our armor,
our reason for holding tight and holding back.
and much of the world will tell us it is too hard,
too ugly, too broken.
this will become *one* narrative, *one* truth.
and yet, in one's lifetime,
so precious and tender,
there will also be endless stories of bridges being built
and that will begin to mend our hearts.
again and again, our shattered insides
will fill with light that pierces through the fractures
and tears down our walls and melts our armor
and gives us our reason for letting go
and moving forward.
and when the world tells us it's too hard,
too ugly, too broken…
we will know both the brutality
and the beauty of humanity
and we will rise anyway.

the ripple

there's a softness coming through.
my **revol**ution isn't led by force, but by love.
my voice isn't loud, but resonate.
my fists aren't up, but rather,
my hands are open and extending.
my ideas may not move mountains,
but they certainly will move a few souls
and the ripple effect - *the ripple*
that's what I'm counting on.

we are women

we are women
we are the ones who *remember*
we are here to bring the medicine
of remembrance.
to awaken those who have fallen asleep
to take the hands of those who feel alone and lost
to touch the hearts of those who have forgotten.
we are the tender, *wild* hearts
whose strong backs
have carried a lifetime
of burdens and blessings.
when it is forgotten
we are here to remind the world
that we are the queens who can birth babies
and birth dreams.
we weep
we build
we restore
we sacrifice
we hold up and we hold on
we…
are women.
and we are the ones who *remember*
we are here to bring the medicine
of remembrance.

love spoke

*a*nd when all felt lost, *love spoke...*

your tender heart is not something to hide away
in fear of its shattering,
for a tender heart is made of *cosmic stuff* -
an explosion doesn't destroy you,
it turns you into a supernova,
and you shine *brighter.*

heartbreak makes room for *even more* love

heartbreak is a growing pain.
it's the heart growing bigger,
stretching, *expanding*
to create capacity
for *even more* love.
be tender with yourself
you're growing, darling.

widening

my hope is simply that you are *widening* your life.
widening it so the breadth and depth of your arms
can hold *all the love* that wants to be held.
i hope you are finding ways to open *up* and open *out*,
so the world can be graced by all your beauty, *within*.
i hope instead of spreading yourself thin,
you have learned to spread your wings wide.
i hope you create space in the minutes of your existence
to move slow,
so you can feel, savor, and experience
how precious it *all* is.
i hope you look in the mirror and fall in love *even more*
with every passing year.
and i hope when your heart hurts,
you still know gratitude,
because you have touched a love so true and beautiful
in *yourself*
that you understand, in your bones,
that the hurt only exists
because love did first.

the path inside of me

i have found the path
that leads me to something
deeper, wider, *wiser.*
a life that feels more
true and beautiful.
for so long
i searched
all the places
outside of me,
where i was told
i would find fulfillment.
only to find
the path was never
over there, or there
but only always,
inside of me.

what do you love?

i love the early mornings when the world falls silent and
i can hear the deepest parts of me singing.

i love the way he looks right into my eyes and holds his
gaze. I almost blush and look away, but instead i stay,
and it's there in each other's gaze, that we *rise* in love,
over and over again.

i love the smell of coffee, cinnamon, and the warmth of a
mug in my bare hands.

i love how even the sun is an artist, casting portraits on
the walls, with shadow and light.

i love color - electric and bold, soft and muted, warm
and rich - it's all so lovely to me.

i love the moments when i feel the world in my heart and
just know in my bones, everything will be ok.

i love the spaces and places my breath takes me.

i love watching children, *be children,* and i love
watching adults be kind and brave, like they did so
naturally when they were children.

i love the smell of a wood burning fire and the sound of
embers crackling.

but most of all…

i love that *love* can so easily be found, even in moments that break our hearts.

what do you love?

for the love of my life (vows to my soul)

i remember lying under the stars in my front yard
making wishes for my future. i was six years old and
even then, maybe more than ever, i could feel your
presence. i don't think i really even knew what that
meant, but here and now, as i reflect on that memory, i
believe i may have known something deeper than words
could have expressed at that time.

i loved sleeping under those stars, feeling so safe and
seen. it felt like i was lying with you under those
magnificent lights - those tiny twinkling punctures in the
universe - the night sky like a dark blanket we could
hide together under. as i felt the stardust in the wiggle of
my toes and in the squint of my eyes, i could sense you.

it's been years since we've spent those nights together
under the stars. and there were moments between then
and now that we didn't connect for sometime. you never
left me - it was alway me who left you (even though it
never felt right - like my bones were hallowed).

i can still feel the brittleness of your absence when i
wouldn't let you in. and every time i came back, with my
head hanging low, you'd be right there waiting for me
with open arms. never judging, never forgetting who i
really was. you have always been 'the one.' *always*. and
so today i kneel before you, with you, within you,
enraptured by you, and forever in awe of your presence,
and i vow to honor you - my sweet love, my compass of

truth, the one i can vulnerably bring all the parts of me
with no judgment, the one who will be with me for all

eternity, forever more, the one that taught me, i am *never*
alone.

this is for you, *my darling soul...*

i vow to remember to breathe slow when i feel lost or
alone, as i know this is the fastest way back to you. and **i
vow** to always find my way back to you, no matter how
far i've wandered off.

i vow to ask, *'does my soul feel safe with this person'*
when i'm exploring new romantic partnerships - to truly
check-in with how 'we' feel in this person's presence.
and if that's not clear, because intimacy can be as
marvelous as it is messy, **i vow** to be vulnerable and
brave in doing what's needed to get to that place with
that person, or move on.

i vow to listen to you daily, to check in with your deepest
curiosities, wishes, and longings for us...as you have
never strayed me wrong. you have always been and will
always be, my compass towards truth.

i vow to not wait for others to delight you, swoon you,
and make you feel special. i'll do it often myself, with
small gestures that light you up, such as buying you
flowers because i know that beauty speaks to you and

flowers remind you to be present to life in a way that you cannot help but to blossom yourself.

i vow to play frank sinatra when you're feeling blue or romantic because i know his words and harmony get under my skin and into *you* in a way that always lift the spirit.

i vow to not sacrifice my connection to you, just to try to prove my worth to another.

i vow to honor your drive and desire for depth in relationship to others and those who can't hang, won't be invited into our world in any significant way.

i vow to believe in you for richer or for poorer, in our mess and in our majesty. and when life gets challenging, i will be by your side, reminding you, what you've always reminded me - that we are larger, better than we know.

i vow to love you for better or for worse. some days we'll be on top of the world and others days we'll feel we want to hide from the world. on either day, you'll still be the light of my life.

i vow to love you in sickness and in health and to see your beauty beyond the stretch marks, cellulite, wrinkles, and bad hair days. i will cuddle you every night, no matter what, for the rest of my life.

And last, but not least…

i vow to have and hold you, respect and see you. and,
most of all, i will love you in a way that you can not help
but to bring forth the best of yourself. and when you feel
messy, weak, rejected, not good enough or worthy...i will
take you outside under the nights sky, tell you to look up,
and we will reminisce on how when i was just six years
old i thought the stars in the sky looked like little cracks
in the universe, and you would wisely, *lovingly* say,
*'that's to remind us that our majesty can be found in our
broken parts.'*

note about this piece: on my 40th birthday (august 4th,
2019), a few months before starting tiny rituals, i created
a ceremony with eight other women after watching a
tedx talk called, 'the person you really need to marry.'
we 'glamped' in nature for a weekend and each married
ourselves in a large belle tent, with each other as
witness. today, i am married to myself and to a
wonderful human named peter. on my left ring finger i
wear a gold ring i gave myself, first, then the ring peter
got me. the ring i got myself is worn first as *a reminder*
of where all love begins - with ourselves. while these
vows were not written as a tiny ritual, they were
certainly a remembrance, and with that i felt deeply
compelled to end the book this way. i offer this practice
up to you, as writing vows to myself has been one of the
most important pieces of writing i have ever written.

CLOSING WORDS

a prayer for remembering

may we all *remember* our true nature
may we pass it down to generations to come
may we let our bones dance it
and the fire of our soul sing it
may we whirl like a whirling dervish until emptied out,
with nothing left, but what is *true*
leaving us humming our essence,
like a chant embedded in the wisdom of our heart
'divine, divine, divine...
i see now, my true nature is,
holy, whole, and wise.'

WITH DEEPEST REVERENCE AND GRATITUDE

First and foremost, a deep bow to that beautiful, creative spirit within that captures us, moves through us, and out of us - creating things we never could have done alone.

Thank you to my yoga students who listened, with so much receptivity and reverence, to my words, and encouraged me to keep writing and to keep sharing. Sometimes people seem braver than they are, so never stop encouraging others - you have no idea how much your encouragement matters.

Thank you Liza Monroy, an incredibly talented writer, loving mother and wife, and a dear friend all the way back from my NYC days. Thank you for reading this book before it was published. Thank you for your generous feedback, your 'blurb' on the back of the book that made me feel so seen, but most of all, thank you for being a steward for the artistry of story-telling and self-expression. You have always held me and others up in their light with such genuine care.

Thank you to my tender, soulful friend, Jennifer McIntosh, for creating such an artistic, soothing home. This book began in your bottom floor sanctuary in 2020 and I attribute my creative spirit being sparked by yours. From the long, languid, deep morning or evening conversations we had, to the somatic release we experienced (dancing, singing, breathwork, running, crying, laughing), your presence in my life inspired some of the most sacred *rememberings* within me.

Thank you to my husband, my rock, and my book formatting king, Peter Lam. Everything in my world, from my he(art) to my community, has become richer since you've been in my life. You bring out the best in me, you are the yin to my yang - keeping me grounded and somewhat patient. You help me *remember* what matters most, and your deep care for me (and what matters to me) has been the greatest gift of my life. I'm honored to *'yes, and'* through this great adventure called life with you. I love you to the moon and back, a million lifetimes over.

Thank you to so many glorious humans that have held me in retreats, classes, workshops, or shared words that have inspired me. These are often the people that don't get acknowledged. These spaces matter - so thank you! Thank you to Nisha Moodley for hosting a retreat in 2017 that brought me back to poetry (you are literal magic). Thank you to Marybeth LaRue for a beautiful virtual workshop in 2021 that revealed to me the most beautiful definition of embodiment - *to be deeply present to direct experience*. This definition landed in my bones and opened portals in me that poured into these pages. Thank you to Tanya Markul for hosting a 30 day journey called Publish Your Poetry that helped me turn these poems into a book, *and,* offered some great prompts that lead to a couple of pieces in these pages.

And last but not least, thank you to all the poets, artists, musicians, and teachers who dare to go into the dark, and make light. You are, and always have been, my greatest inspiration.

ABOUT THE AUTHOR

Amber Campion is an international mindfulness-based yoga teacher, speaker, and writer working at the intersection of embodiment and leadership. Her deepest dharma is to be a light for people to bring their *full* self to the world. She's taught yoga, mindfulness, and integrative leadership everywhere from the inside of prisons to deep in the jungle, and is known for facilitating *real* experiences... *imperfections* included.

www.ingramcontent.com/pod-product-compliance
Lightning Source LLC
Chambersburg PA
CBHW051309250726
48656CB00004B/1571